IMPROVING THE FOOD ENVIRONMENT
THROUGH NUTRITION STANDARDS:
A GUIDE FOR GOVERNMENT PROCUREMENT

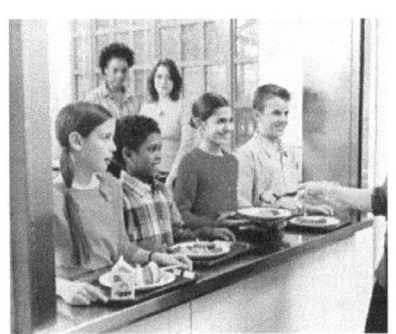
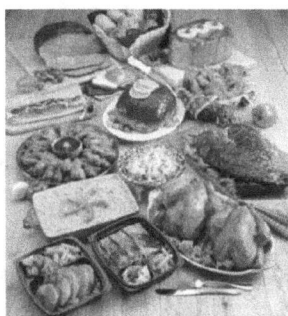
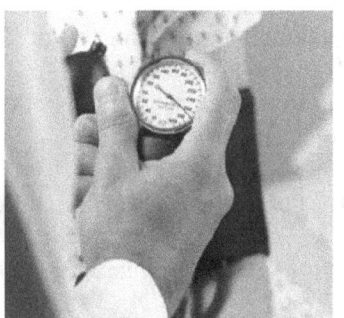
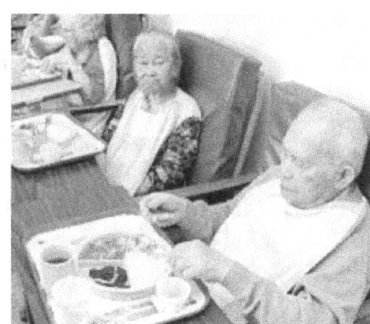

National Center for Chronic Disease Prevention and Health Promotion
Division for Heart Disease and Stroke Prevention

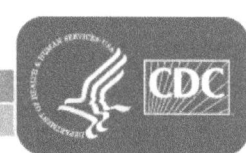

Acknowledgments

CDC would like to thank all those who provided input during the development of *Improving the Food Environment Through Nutrition Standards: A Guide for Government Procurement.*

Primary contributors:

Jessica M. Lee, MS, RD, LD
Division for Heart Disease and Stroke Prevention
National Center for Chronic Disease Prevention and Health Promotion
Centers for Disease Control and Prevention

Janelle Peralez Gunn, MPH, RD
Division for Heart Disease and Stroke Prevention
National Center for Chronic Disease Prevention and Health Promotion
Centers for Disease Control and Prevention

Lauren Gase, MPH, CHES
Office of the Director
Office of the Associate Director for Policy
Centers for Disease Control and Prevention

Nicole Blair, MPH
Division for Heart Disease and Stroke Prevention
National Center for Chronic Disease Prevention and Health Promotion
Centers for Disease Control and Prevention

Additional support and valuable input came from:

Staff in the Centers for Disease Control and Prevention's Division for Heart Disease and Stroke Prevention and Public Health Law Program

Participants in CDC's 2010 Public Health Law Summit on Sodium Reduction

Special acknowledgment is given to the following for their assistance in the development of this guide:

Staff in the Bureau of Chronic Disease Prevention and Control of the New York City Department of Health and Mental Hygiene

Marice Ashe, JD, MPH
Public Health Law & Policy

Contents

Suggested citation:

Centers for Disease Control and Prevention. *Improving the Food Environment Through Nutrition Standards: A Guide for Government Procurement.* U.S. Department of Health and Human Services, Centers for Disease Control and Prevention, National Center for Chronic Disease Prevention and Health Promotion, Division for Heart Disease and Stroke Prevention. February 2011.

For online materials: www.cdc.gov/salt.

Purpose and Intended Use

Improving the Food Environment Through Nutrition Standards: A Guide for Government Procurement provides practical guidance to states and localities for use when developing, adopting, implementing, and evaluating a food procurement policy. For the purposes of this Guide, the term "food procurement policy" refers to a policy officially adopted by a state or local government (or a state or local government agency) requiring that the food it purchases, provides, or makes available contains key nutrients at levels that do not exceed standards established by public health authorities. Such a policy might, for example, define the maximum amount of sodium allowed in foods purchased, contracted for, or served by a day care center run with city dollars. In addition, procurement policies use the purchasing power of government to make an impact on food availability and add to the overall demand for more healthful products. Procurement policies can model healthier food environments, potentially drive the reformulation of foods, and have an impact on diverse settings (e.g., employee cafeterias, correctional facilities, schools, child care centers, public hospitals, senior centers, parks).

- Food procurement policies should be comprehensive and include standards for a variety of food components such as sodium, trans fat, and sugar.
- From a purchasing perspective, having such a policy means considering not only the cost and quality of products but also the overall healthfulness of each food purchased. How much sodium does it have? Is it free of industrially produced trans fat?
- As a practical matter, the procurement policy requires seeking healthful foods that will contribute to more nutritious environments and healthful diets.

Why Focus on the Food Environment?

According to the United States Department of Agriculture, food consumption in the United States has increased by 16 percent since 1970, corresponding to an increased calorie intake from 2,234 calories per person per day in 1970 to 2,757 calories in 2003.[1] In addition, a study from 2003 found significant changes in portion sizes, with portion sizes ranging from an increase of 49 to 133 calories per item among commonly consumed foods such as salty snacks, soft drinks, hamburgers, French fries, and Mexican food.[2]

Compared to the early 1900s, today's U.S. food supply has, per person, 35% more sodium than it did in the early 1900s due to the availability of more processed foods.[3] There also are more fat and sweeteners per capita in today's food supply than there were at the beginning of the 20th century, translating to nearly 30% of energy intake of the U.S. population being derived from nutrient-poor foods, including soft drinks, salty snacks, sweets, and desserts.[4] A recent Institute of Medicine report, *Strategies to Reduce Sodium Intake in the United States,* recommended as a supporting strategy that "food retailers, governments, businesses, institutions, and other large-scale organizations that purchase or distribute food establish sodium specifications for the foods they purchase and the food operators they oversee."[5] Such procurement policies, if comprehensive, will support an improvement in the healthfulness of the food supply and decreased intake of nutrients of concern, generally.

---

[1] Hodan Farah H, Buzby J. U.S. food consumption up 16 percent since 1970. *Amber Waves.* 2005;3:5.

[2] Nielson S, Popkin B. Patterns and trends in food portion sizes, 1977–1998. *JAMA.* 2003;289(4):450–453. doi: 10.1001/jama.289.4.450.

[3] Gerrior S, Bente L. Nutrient content of the U.S. food supply, 1909–99: a summary report. Home Economics Research Report No. 55. Washington, DC: U.S. Department of Agriculture, Center for Nutrition Policy and Promotion; 2002.

[4] Block G. Foods contributing to energy intake in the US: data from NHANES III and NHANES 1999–2000. *J Food Composition Analysis.* 2004;17:439–447.

[5] Institute of Medicine. *Strategies to reduce sodium intake in the United States.* Washington, DC: National Academies; 2010.

According to the 2010 *Dietary Guidelines for Americans*, eating and physical activity patterns that are focused on consuming fewer calories, making informed food choices, and being physically active can help people attain and maintain a healthy weight, reduce their risk of chronic disease, and promote overall health. Select key recommendations of the 2010 Dietary Guidelines include:

- Reduce daily sodium intake to less than 2,300 milligrams (mg) and further reduce intake to 1,500 mg among persons who are 51 and older and those of any age who are African American or have hypertension, diabetes, or chronic kidney disease. The 1,500 mg recommendation applies to about half of the U.S. population, including children, and the majority of adults.[6] Yet on average, Americans consume significantly more sodium than these limits—more than 3,400 mg per day.[7]
- Consume less than 10 percent of calories from saturated fatty acids by replacing them with monounsaturated and polyunsaturated fatty acids.
- Consume less than 300 mg per day of dietary cholesterol.
- Keep trans fatty acid consumption as low as possible by limiting foods that contain synthetic sources of trans fats, such as partially hydrogenated oils, and by limiting other solid fats.
- Reduce the intake of calories from solid fats and added sugars.
- Limit the consumption of foods that contain refined grains, especially refined grain foods that contain solid fats, added sugars, and sodium.

State and local agencies can be critical players in transforming the food system to help slow rising rates of disease, such as coronary heart disease and stroke, which are related to the consumption of foods high in fat and salt, the latter of which is found in most processed foods in excess. Such agencies can make a difference by modeling healthful nutrition and adopting food purchasing policies and practices in their own facilities that promote healthful food in line with the Dietary Guidelines for Americans recommendations. In turn, procurement policies for purchasing and providing healthful foods can contribute to improving the health of not only the citizens served by city and state agencies but also their employees.

Section I: Introduction

Section Overview:
- Where can a procurement policy be established?
- Benefits of a sound food procurement policy.
- Importance of complementary efforts.

Establishing a procurement policy is a doable, viable, and feasible strategy for state and local governments to put your money where your mouth is. Establishing a procurement policy is one strategy that can be undertaken to support healthful changes to foods that are offered, served, and consumed and will complement other strategies and efforts. Some governments and organizations already have standards related to the foods they offer and serve. For instance, the Department of Health and Human Services developed worksite guidance affecting food served in Federal cafeterias and through vending machines (details can be found in Appendix A).

---

[6] U.S. Department of Agriculture and U.S. Department of Health and Human Services. *Dietary guidelines for Americans, 2010.* 7th edition. Washington, DC: Government Printing Office; 2010.

[7] U.S. Department of Agriculture. What we eat in America. Available from: http://www.ars.usda.gov/SP2UserFiles/Place/12355000/pdf/0506/usual_nutrient_intake_sodium_2003-06.pdf.

Comprehensive food procurement policies were recently introduced via an executive order in New York City and by the state of Massachusetts (see Appendix A for some examples of procurement standards). A food procurement policy may be implemented in different settings and venues. For example, the establishment of such a policy or changes to existing policies can be made by:

- State and local governments.
- School systems.
- Work sites.
- Hospitals.
- Institutionalized populations (e.g., those in nursing homes or correctional facilities).
- Assisted living communities.
- Colleges and universities.
- Community-based organizations (including faith-based organizations).
- Day care centers.

The intended audience for this Guide is **state and local governments.** A state or local government procurement policy can have an impact on a variety of settings, including work sites, areas served through distributive food programs (e.g., a meals program for seniors), day care centers, schools, prisons, probation camps, and concession stands operated by the jurisdiction. It is important to remember that what works for one setting in a jurisdiction may not be appropriate for another. For instance, a school setting may require different procurement standards than a prison would, and it may also require a different implementation plan. This is not to say that one can't apply the same nutritional standards to one's entire jurisdiction; rather, it is important to ascertain the appropriateness and acceptability of those standards in the various settings that will be affected by them. You may want to establish a baseline standard for all, and then further refine the standards for specific populations as needed, based on age, health status, or other considerations.

A successful food procurement policy will be fully integrated with the overall goals and objectives of the setting in which it is carried out. It will clearly state the setting's goals, identify procurement strategies, and commit resources to those strategies. It will also set targets and timelines and establish means for evaluating progress and making adjustments (for instance, if new dietary guidelines are released and the standards need to be updated).

The information contained in this Guide will help you consider the breadth of settings where you may be able to influence food procurement, the relevant organizational and policy constraints, and the factors you will want to consider, including a checklist of key decisions, to help develop and implement a successful food procurement policy.

Potential Benefits of a Sound Food Procurement Policy

Food procurement policies can be designed to make healthier food more readily available, affordable, and appealing. These policies can work to change individual factors (e.g., knowledge of how to choose healthy options), social factors (e.g., social norms), and environmental factors (e.g., access to healthy options). Food procurement polices use existing food dollars to create a more nutritious food environment and drive demand toward increased availability and demand for more healthful products.

Food procurement policies can target many nutrients and set standards for calories, fat, trans fat, and sugar to increase the overall healthfulness of food options and provide a more healthful food environment. Procurement policies change the role of state and local government from a passive consumer to an active driver of the market, in the process providing greater demand for and access to healthful foods.

Although the focus of this document is on comprehensive food procurement policies, Figure I depicts as an example how the potential elements of a food procurement policy may work to influence individual, social, environmental, and biological factors to reduce sodium consumption and produce improved health outcomes such as decreased blood pressure and associated morbidity and mortality.

Figure I. Potential benefits related to reduced sodium consumption from implementing a food procurement policy.

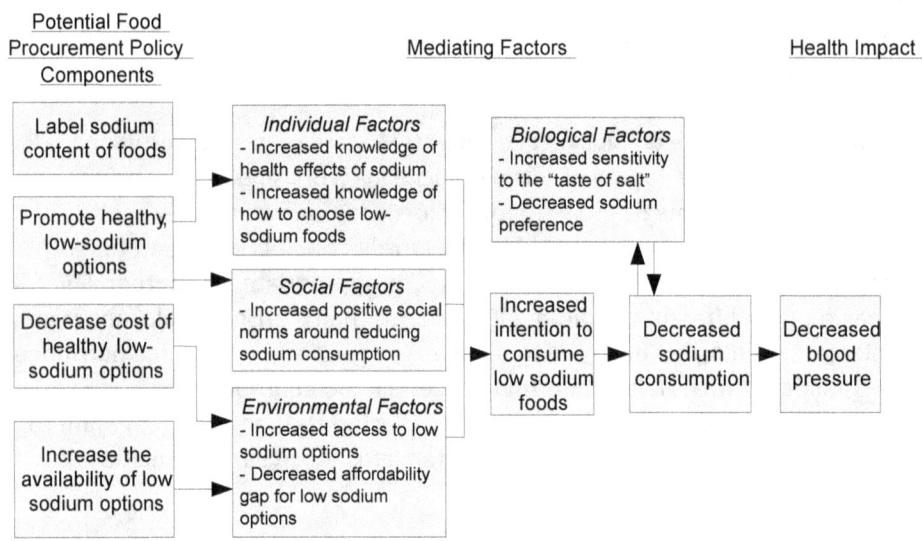

Additional benefits of the procurement of healthful food by state and local agencies may include:
- Contributing to the organizational mission (health departments).
- Avoiding negative publicity associated with purchasing unhealthful products.
- Setting a positive example for constituents, employees, stakeholders, or other employers.
- Building awareness and support among decision makers, budget holders, and purchasing staff.
- Facilitating communication with suppliers, purchasers, employees, and the public.
- Increasing consumer demand for healthier food from food suppliers (see Appendix B on how to increase consumer demand).
- Reducing the large economic burden of health care costs associated with heart disease, stroke, heart attack, and heart and kidney failure.

Procurement: More than a Stand-Alone Policy

Implementing a food procurement policy represents a potentially effective component of a **comprehensive strategy** to reduce sodium and eliminate trans fat consumption and improve nutrition broadly. Cafeterias and other settings run by government often provide only a fraction of their clients' daily food intake, limiting the potential impact of an improved food environment to these settings. To create a food environment in line with the current *Dietary Guidelines for Americans* recommendations, a variety of strategies will likely be needed, such as those that increase access to affordable healthful foods in the community or add to individuals' knowledge of healthier food choices and motivations to try them. Increasing consumption of unprocessed foods, such as fresh fruits and vegetables, will further improve nutritional intake by replacing foods that contain nutrients of concern with more healthful choices that are high in vitamins, minerals, and other essential nutrients.

Often, state and local jurisdictions are large purchasers of food. Directing more of these dollars toward foods that meet minimum nutritional requirements—and away from foods that don't—will demonstrate increased demand for more healthful foods. State and local action can also complement national efforts to influence both food quality and food supply.

Section II: Policy Development

Section Overview:
- Building the team.
- Assessing the food environment.
- Conducting a needs assessment.
- Assessing opportunities and barriers.

The development of a procurement policy should incorporate a participatory approach. Including key individuals and groups near the beginning of the process may help to increase buy-in and, later, facilitate implementation of the policy. Steps taken by you to determine jurisdiction (authority to act) and assess opportunities and barriers can assist in determining the range and scope your policy will contain.

Building the Team

Some communities have active coalitions and leadership teams focused on preventing chronic disease risk factors. These existing assets should be utilized wherever possible. If a new team needs to be formed, the team should be built early in the procurement process, ideally at the very beginning. The first step is to identify potential core team members, who may include:
- Public health department staff.
- Staff from other offices or departments who will implement the policy or be affected by it.
- Organization management.
- A representative of the executive office.

In addition, you may want to consider forming a larger workgroup or advisory committee. Identify others whom you will need on your side to develop, adopt, and implement the policy. Specifically, consider involving:
- Food contractors or food service vendors.
- Grantees or subcontractors of your jurisdiction that provide food.
- Health impact assessment (HIA) workers.

In addition, consider champions and partners that can serve as allies in moving your policy forward. Specifically, reach out to:
- Coalitions, groups, or advocacy organizations that focus on or benefit from improving the food environment.
- Representatives of sub-populations experiencing the highest burden of high blood pressure.
- Representatives of health-disparate populations.
- Work-site wellness committees.
- Unions.
- Insurance companies that provide wellness-related benefits to the jurisdiction's employees.

- Dietitians or nutritionists on staff within the organization.
- Nutrition programs and health educators.
- Clinicians such as physicians, nurses, therapists, and other professionals.
- Hospitals in your jurisdiction.

Assessing the Food Environment: Where Is Food Purchased, Distributed, or Served?

During the policy development phase, the food environment will need to be assessed to determine where food is purchased, distributed, or served within your jurisdiction. Often, jurisdictions have a number of different departments, agencies, or offices that are involved with the purchase, distribution, or vending of food. Understanding the total scope of opportunity to improve the food environment will help determine the potential impact of the policy and what range of actions may be taken. When assessing the food environment, it also is important to consider pursuing a jurisdiction-wide policy rather than working site by site or agency by agency. Jurisdiction-wide policies will maximize public health impact and provide more healthful food for your buck.

Some settings that purchase, serve, sell, distribute, or contract out their food service include:
- Work-site cafeterias.
- Work-site vending machines.
- Distributive meal programs (e.g., senior meals, after-school snacks).
- Institutionalized populations (e.g., people in prisons or probation camps).
- Child care facilities (e.g., day care centers).
- Schools.
- Recreational facilities (e.g., museums, golf courses, parks, pools).
- Concession stands (e.g., snack shops).
- Meetings or conferences hosted or funded within the jurisdiction.
- Hospitals.

Considering this range of settings, you may also want to assess:
- How many meals and snacks does each setting serve?
- To whom do these settings serve food (i.e., what is the patron profile)?
- Where are these settings located?
- Do these settings prepare (cook) their own food, or do they contract their food services to an outside entity?
- Do these settings have subcontractors or grantees?

Existing nutrition policies. During this process, consider similar existing initiatives currently under way where procurement standards could be worked into the language, including policies in other jurisdictions. Assessing policies in other jurisdictions will determine where states or communities can utilize the same standards and requirements. Doing so will assist in streamlining requirements and align a larger market share, thus encouraging the food industry to make changes in their food. For example, if the 50 largest school districts had the same procurement policy standards, they would have a large impact on the food environment and on availability of and access to healthful food. In addition, check to see if there are any nutrition policies or standards already in place. Consider programs that distribute food, such as meals to seniors or after-school snacks. If you are working at the state level, consider entities, such as cities or counties, to which you provide funding for programs or institutions that serve food, such as schools or prisons. An effective way to do this is to release a call for work or something similar requesting that all settings in your jurisdiction provide background if they have a similar policy in place. Describe what you are looking for and ask the departments to report to you on what exists in their area.

Consider assessing the existence of the following types of policies (and adherence to these policies):
- Healthy vending.
- Guidelines or nutrition standards for gatherings (conferences, meetings, parties, etc.).
- Guidelines for nutrition standards for cafeterias or lunch rooms.
- Menu labeling.
- Work-site wellness.

As described above, you may be able to build on existing policies. For each setting, you will want to determine:
- What nutrition standards are being used by the department, program, or food service setting?
- What settings do these policies and standards cover?
- Are they voluntary or mandatory standards?
- What has been the level of compliance and adherence to the standards?
- What barriers or facilitators exist to meeting existing standards and policies?
- What lessons have been learned from implementing these standards and policies?

Conducting a Needs Assessment

The next step is to conduct a needs assessment to help you better understand the food environment and determine potential opportunities and barriers relative to the implementation of a policy.

Determining where you have jurisdiction. After you have determined the settings in which food is purchased, distributed, or served, the next step is to assess where you have control—essentially, where you can change the nutrition standards or procurement policies. The ability to set policies or determine the substance of a policy will depend on whether you have jurisdiction (authority) and on your understanding of that authority. For example, if federal standards apply, as in reimbursable school meals, are the standards a "floor" (i.e., they require you to meet certain criteria but allow specific policies to go further) or a "ceiling" (i.e., specific policies cannot be more rigorous than the standards)? For each department, program, or food service setting, consider:
- Who sets or determines the standards for this department, program, or food service setting (federal or state government, the contracting process, the employee purchaser)?
- For which settings can you set or strengthen standards for foods purchased, served, or sold?
- For which settings can you influence the setting or strengthening of standards for foods purchased, served, or sold? (For example, can you do this in museum cafeterias that are run in partnership with the museum foundation and the city?)
- Whose approval is needed to set or strengthen standards (e.g., mayor, city council, school board, department head, county commissioners)?
- How is approval granted?
- What is the process for getting a policy approved?

If there are various standards and policies across agencies in your jurisdiction, consider how these policies could be streamlined into a jurisdiction-wide policy for larger health impact.

Defining the contract process. Likely, the venues and agencies identified on page 6 use different contractors and different contract procedures for food materials and food services. You will want to assess the current process for contracting in each agency that is identified. Potential questions include:

- How many vendors or contractors does your jurisdiction currently work with?
- What is the process for selecting a contractor?
- What factors are important for selection?
    - During the selection process, how much weight is placed on the ability of the contractor to meet the nutrition standards that have been set forth?
- How often are contracts renegotiated?
- Would the existing contractors(s) be willing and able to meet defined nutrient standards?
    - Do they already offer "healthy meals" programs? (Many do!)
- Are you able to solicit new contractors?
- Are you able to change contractors if they cannot meet new standards (e.g., by giving them "first right of refusal")?
- Can the current contracts be amended prior to expiration?

The Logistics of a Needs Assessment

Whom do I ask? Depending on the types of questions you need answered, you will want to include the following types of people in the needs assessment:

- Departments that purchase, distribute, or serve food (i.e., those that will be affected by the policy).
    - Contract managers and food purchasers.
    - Nutritionists and dietitians.
    - Grantees and subcontractors.
    - Food service vendors.
    - Food service staff (such as those who prepare the food).
    - Vending machine contractors.
- Those who will have to pass the policy.
- Those who will have to implement and oversee the policy.
- Those who have already implemented procurement policies.

How do I ask? This needs assessment can be conducted by administering a survey or by interviewing stakeholders. Although it is often less time-consuming to conduct a survey, if you have time, we suggest that you **interview stakeholders** either in person or by phone. Conducting these interviews will provide you with a deeper understanding of some of the opportunities you will have as well as the barriers to implementing the policy. In addition, conducting interviews will allow you to start building a relationship with those individuals who will have to pass, implement, or enforce the policy and create buy-in among those persons. Furthermore, during interviews you can help answer any questions that individuals might have.

How can I use this information? Data gathered from this assessment will help you in deciding:

- How to work with policy makers.
- Which settings you will need to work with (and how you will need to work with them) to implement the policy.
- What kinds of nutrition standards are realistic and feasible.
- How much it will cost you to implement the policy (e.g., what further staff and training is needed).

In addition, the needs assessment can serve as a baseline assessment (a snapshot of where you are starting from), which could be a useful source of data for your program's evaluation. You may want to collect specific data during the needs assessment that will provide you with needed information that can help you answer your evaluation questions (see Section V: Evaluation: Measuring Progress).

Assessing Opportunities and Barriers

An important next step is to assess the potential opportunities to implement a procurement policy in the settings of interest and the barriers to implementation. The needs assessment will provide you with critical insight into how you will develop the policy. When seeking to understand opportunities and barriers, consider the following.

Where is there appropriate staff in place?
- Which departments have experts in nutrition (dietitians, nutritionists, etc.)?
- Which departments have certified purchasing experts?
- Which departments have health or wellness educators?
- What other staff can serve as "champions" for policy implementation?

What are the attitudes and level of knowledge about nutrition?
- To what extent is the nutrition content of the food a priority?
- Are departments or decision makers concerned about the healthfulness of foods they offer or that their employees consume?
- Do department representatives or decision makers think it is feasible to improve the food environment? Why or why not?

Where is there major support for or resistance to the proposed policy?
- How feasible do you think it would be to implement a policy or strategy that strengthened or set nutrition standards?
  - How might such a policy affect your organization and your work?
  - How easy or difficult do you think it would be to manage and enforce this policy?
  - What would be some benefits of implementing such a policy?
  - Whom do we need to have "on board" to implement this policy? Who would be some of the major supporters?
  - What barriers might be faced in implementing this policy or strategy? How might these barriers be overcome? (For a list of potential barriers, see Appendix B.)
- What support would the policy have if approached from particular angles, such as environmental reasons, prevention of obesity, and economic benefits for local farms and companies?

Section III: Policy Adoption

Section Overview:
- Modes of policy adoption.
- Considering the language of the policy.

Food procurement policies can be adopted through a variety of official means; among them are statutes, ordinances, administrative regulations, executive orders, and other formal statements. These procurement policies may apply to food that is purchased by a government or agency, provided to the employees of a government or agency by contracted vendors (e.g., in agency cafeterias), made available for purchase from vending machines to employees and members of the public who are visiting government facilities, or provided to clients and other people who use services supported by a government or agency (e.g., children enrolled in day care programs maintained for an agency's employees, students in public schools and universities, residents and inmates in state institutions). The policies may also apply to food in other settings where a government or agency has an official role.

The adoption of policy will ideally be spearheaded by the procurement champion who was identified when the team was built. What it takes to adopt a procurement policy will vary from place to place depending on the jurisdiction. A procurement policy can go into effect from an executive order by a mayor or governor, or a policy can be adopted via an ordinance or regulatory body, such as a school board, city council, or county commission.

Know the process in your jurisdiction, and determine how a policy needs to be adopted for your particular jurisdiction, as there may be more than one way. If there is more than one route, determine the most feasible and promising route to adopt the policy. If you learned in Assessing the Food Environment that nutrition or health-related policies, standards, legislation, etc., have previously been adopted in your jurisdiction, it may be easiest to adopt the procurement policy through the route that was followed in those cases. Considerations include:
- Who would send a draft executive order to the mayor?
- How are new regulations and policies introduced?
- Who needs to introduce the policy?

Finally, consider communications that would support the policy. In terms of information, you may want to provide:
- Relevant state data (and local data, if available) on poor nutrition, the overconsumption of nutrients of concern, and the burden of high blood pressure, high cholesterol, and cardiovascular disease in your jurisdiction.
- The potential reach, as well as impact on health, food costs, and productivity, of implementing the policy.
- The potential costs and the resources needed to implement the policy.

Finally, consider the timing of other related policy actions as well as key meetings and other good opportunities for presenting information.

Considering the Language of the Policy
When developing language that will be included in the policy, consider language that will ensure that the potential public health impact of the policy will be maximized. This can be done by addressing the broadest possible reach and coverage in the policy language and prescribing the policy across the jurisdiction. To aid with implementation, the following elements should be **clearly defined** in the policy's language:
- Which departments, programs, or food service settings will be required to implement the policy, and which entities, if any, will be exempt?
  - Consider their source of funding when making this determination. For example, make it clear that even if entities are funded with federal dollars, they are required to implement the policy that your jurisdiction is implementing.
  - Use information gathered from your needs assessment to help determine which entities will be exempt. For example, in both the Massachusetts and New York City policies,

concessions were not included among affected foods served by city agencies and vending, initially.
- o Consider how the policy will apply to catering and conferences.
- o Consider whether the standards can be applied only to "formal" purchases, or if they can be applied to informal settings where food is served, such as office parties and meetings.
- Who will oversee implementation of the policy, and who will enforce it?
  - o Implementation and enforcement might not be handled by the same person or agency.
- What is the timeline for implementation?
  - o Will departments, programs, or food service settings be required to implement the standards within a defined time frame? Will they be required to implement all the standards at once, or will they be phased in?
  - o What is the timing for renewing all affected contracts?
- What are the penalties for noncompliance?
  - o What will happen if departments, programs, or food service settings do not comply with the policy? Establishing penalties may be one way to ensure that settings do comply.
- Which nutrition standards should be included? In determining these standards, consider the following questions:
  - o Will you set your own standards or use preexisting standards?
    - ▪ If you are considering preexisting standards, you must also consider whether they are appropriate for that particular audience. (For example, an elementary school may have different nutrient standards than would an adult correctional facility.)
  - o Will the standards be phased in (continuing to be refined and made more stringent over time) or set forth just once?
  - o Will the standards be piloted in one venue before their use is expanded to all agencies in the jurisdiction?
  - o Will the standards be tailored to each department, program, or food service setting, or will they be the same for every setting in your jurisdiction?
    - ▪ You will need to consider the variety of needs and populations served by each agency and whether uniform standards will be appropriate.
  - o Will standards be defined for categories of food items (e.g., milk, meats, cheeses, snacks) or for total meal allowances (e.g., a standard of one-third of the recommended daily sodium or saturated fat allowance for the lunch meal)?
    - ▪ The standards may differ according to the venue. A work-site cafeteria may want to adopt individual food standards, whereas in a setting such as a nursing home or correctional facility (where everyone is served the same meal), standards may be set per meal or per day (e.g., a daily limit of 1,500 or 2,300 mg sodium). See Box I for an example.
  - o Can the settings meet the standards in the beginning, or will you need to allow time to catch up?
    - ▪ It may not be feasible for suppliers and distributors to meet all the standards right away. If this is the case, you will need to consider allowing for more stringent standards over time.
- Other nutrition issues to consider:
  - o Is the policy focused on adding healthier options to the menu (e.g., fruits and vegetables, whole grains), restricting unhealthy options, or both?

- o Are you setting new standards or reformulating existing options (e.g., by reducing sodium, sugars, saturated fats, and trans fats or by decreasing calories and portion sizes)?
- o What other complementary policies, such as menu labeling and pricing strategies, can encourage healthy eating?

Box I. Example of standards: New York City

> The New York City Agency Food Standards require all individual items to have 480 mg or less sodium per serving, but also sets lower standards for certain food groups, such as breads, cereals, vegetables, and canned and frozen seafood. These standards may apply to all foods purchased and served at the facility. New York City has standards for individual foods, as well as for meals and snacks served in locations that serve one to three meals per day.

Draw from the data that you gathered during your needs assessment when considering what policy language will work best in your jurisdiction. Consider what is feasible based on:
- The number and types of settings that serve food and the baseline nutrient levels of this food.
- The willingness of key decision makers to pass the policy.
- The resources, including staffing, that you have available for implementation and enforcement of the policy (see Section IV).
- Feasibility of making changes to the policy language at a later date. Once a policy is in place, it may be difficult to go back later and make it more stringent.

Section IV: Implementation

Section Overview:
- Determining the resources needed for implementation.
- Working with the settings that must implement the policy.
- Ensuring compliance with the policy.

Obtaining the necessary support for implementing a procurement policy is a key to its success. This should include designating a point of contact within each department or food service setting and identifying and communicating with allies. The timeline that was developed during the planning stage will need to be clearly communicated to all parties, and an evaluation plan will need to be developed.

Determining the Resources Needed for Implementation

When developing a procurement policy, you should consider how much it will cost to implement. Determining the costs up front can help you decide how much funding is needed and what level of funding you need to communicate to decision makers. There are a number of costs to consider that can be roughly estimated by assigning costs to the resources described below. Implementation may vary across the jurisdiction for agencies with differing sub-populations.

Staffing. Staff will be needed to assist with a range of issues, including overseeing implementation of the policy, providing training and technical assistance to agencies on how to meet the standards, and tracking whether agencies are complying with the standards. Staff may be needed at three different levels: (1) within the agency (e.g., the New York City food policy coordinator is located in the mayor's office); (2) in the department responsible for coordinating implementation of the policy (e.g., Department of Public Health); and (3) within each of the departments or offices required to implement the policy (e.g., Office of Education, Department of Parks and Recreation). Possible staff positions at each of these levels are described in Table 1.

Table 1. Potential staff needed to implement a food procurement policy.

Level			Estimated
Agency	Food policy coordinator	• Ensure that each agency is complying with the policy and administer penalties for noncompliance. • Liaise with the regulating body. • Coordinate all food-related policy and environmental initiatives across the agency.	25%–100%
Coordinating department	Project coordinator	• Oversee and coordinate implementation efforts. • Plan trainings, develop materials, and design and implement monitoring and evaluation systems.	50%–100%
	Policy analyst	• Plan trainings, provide technical assistance, and develop training materials. • Ensure compliance of menus and products with standards. • Conduct evaluation.	25%–100%
	Training coordinator	• Assess training needs. • Plan, develop, and deliver trainings.	10%–50%
	Nutritionist/ registered dietitian	• Provide expertise on nutrition-related issues. • Plan trainings and provide technical assistance on how to meet the standards. • Help ensure compliance of menus and products with standards.	25%–50%

Department/ office	Department coordinator(s)	• Serve as a point of contact for each agency that has to implement the policy.
		• Work with the agency to:
		  ○ Plan the menu.
		  ○ Establish contracts.
		• Provide technical assistance to agency grantees or contractors.
		• Ensure compliance of the agency with the standards.
			10%–25% per department

You will likely be able to draw on existing staff to help fill these positions. For example, if a department already has a dietitian on staff, that person may be able to use some of his or her time to help implement the new standards. Some positions may be combined (e.g., the training coordinator and policy analyst may be one person). **At minimum**, for the first year of policy development and implementation, it is important to have each of the following:
- Food policy coordinator (at least 25%).
- Project coordinator (100%).
- Nutritionist or registered dietitian (at least 50%).

Needs for staffing may decrease over time as monitoring systems are established, staff is trained, and departments and vendors become better able to meet the standards.

Training and technical assistance. Resources will most likely have to be budgeted for training. The needs for training will depend on the audience, their current level of knowledge, and the complexity of the standards.

Costs of food. Potentially significant costs to consider are those for extra foods purchased after implementing the policy (e.g., in switching from unhealthy to healthier foods). Some changes may be cost-neutral, however, such as a switch from whole milk to skim milk. In contrast, a switch from canned to fresh vegetables or the purchase of low-sodium specialty items may involve increased costs up front. These costs will likely decrease over time, however, as more low-sodium options are made available in the food marketplace.

To estimate these costs, begin by investigating potential changes in your menus or purchasing with your current food contractors or vendors. Often, large food vendors have existing healthy options that they can offer at little or no increased cost. Also, work with purchasing agents or consider group purchasing organizations to help negotiate lower prices. If different jurisdictions work together, pooled leverage and purchasing power is created, thus helping to lower the cost of food.

Consider your current food budget to determine if an acute increase in food costs in the short term could be withstood. What would a 1%, 5%, or 10% increase in the cost of food mean? A short-term increase in food costs could create cost savings in the long term with decreased accesses to nutrient-poor foods and increased access to health-promoting foods.

Working with the Settings That Must Implement the Policy

Designate a point of contact in each department, program, or food service setting. To facilitate implementation of the policy, it is important to designate a point of contact or a champion in each setting who is required to implement the policy. Each point of contact should understand and accept the importance of the procurement policy and be willing and able to facilitate its implementation. These points of contact should have personal or professional interests in the policy, and the positions they hold in their organizations and their particular skills should allow them to advocate for the effort and take a leadership role in its implementation. If possible, you should recruit individuals with existing expertise in nutrition or contract management.

The points of contact should be able to dedicate 10%–25% of their time to the procurement policy. Each of them will:
- Serve as a point of contact for communications.
- Work with the setting to plan its menus or allowable options and establish the necessary contracts.
- Provide technical assistance to grantees or contractors.
- Ensure compliance of the setting with the standards.

Look for new allies and foster positive relationships. The move to purchasing healthful foods is not done alone—as you saw in the needs assessment phase, cooperation is needed from a number of players. It is important throughout the process to facilitate an atmosphere of open communication and teamwork. Continue to foster positive relationships with all players, and look for allies inside and outside the government. Food vendors, service providers, and other for-profit and nonprofit partners may have the knowledge and resources to help facilitate implementation.

Develop trainings for different audiences. It is likely that many audiences will need to be trained. Departments, programs, and food service settings will need to be briefed on the policy, its importance, and what specifically they need to do to comply with the policy. The first step is to define the audiences that need to be trained.

Next, you will want to assess what each audience wants (and needs) to know. Trainings for different audiences will vary based on their information needs and their baseline (starting) level of knowledge (see Table 2).

Table 2. Potential audiences and their training needs.

Potential Audience	Training Needs

Cooks/food preparers	• Why proper nutrition is important (health impact).
	• How to prepare healthful foods.
	    ○ Salt substitutes (e.g., herbs and spices in place of salt).
	    ○ Healthful recipes.
	    ○ Cooking techniques.

Food service managers	• Their role in ensuring compliance with the policy (e.g., what the standards "mean" for their food service setting). • The importance of the policy.
Contracts/grants managers or procurement officers	• How to write contract language that complies with the policy. • How to work with grantees in implementing the policy. • Purchasing food and items that meet the standards (what to look for to ensure that the foods purchased are in compliance with the standards). • Purchasing foods at low prices (contract negotiation).
Senior managers	• Their role in ensuring compliance with the policy. • What needs to be reported. • The importance of the policy.

Develop resources. You will want to consider what resources you can develop (see the list below) to help supplement your trainings. By providing people with such resources, you can help illustrate your message and prevent yourself from answering the same questions over and over again. To determine which resources are needed in your jurisdiction, you may want to assess the audience's needs for information, perhaps after a training session.

Potential resources include:
- Standard contract language that departments, programs, or food service settings can tailor to meet their needs.
- Lists of food items (examples) that meet the standards and are acceptable.
- Healthful recipe books.
- Procedures for cooking with less sodium (could be listed on a poster or pocket card).
- Labels and menu boards.
- Educational and promotional materials.
- Visual timeline for implementation.

- Visual depictions of the standards (e.g., food pyramids or guides).
- "One-pagers."
    - *Questions to Ask Your Food Service Vendor or Contractor*
    - *10 Reasons Why a Procurement Policy Is Important*
    - *Communicating the Standards to Grantees*

Ensuring Compliance

The coordinating department (or the agency responsible for ensuring compliance) will need to develop a plan for how compliance processes will be implemented and should communicate this plan to other departments. The policy should have been clearly defined regarding who will oversee policy enforcement and the penalties for noncompliance (see "Considering the Language of the Policy" above). In developing a plan for ensuring compliance, consider:
- Who will ensure compliance?
    - Will each department be responsible for reporting information?
    - Will the coordinating department provide oversight?
- Which departments or programs will be required to submit to the coordinating department?
- What will they be required to submit?
    - Examples include planned menus, nutrient analyses of the menus, and lists of purchased products.
- How often will review occur?
    - Monthly, yearly, each new cycle of menu planning?
- Who will be responsible for administering penalties?
    - How will data be communicated to this agency?

Section V: Evaluation: Measuring Progress

Section Overview:
- Monitoring and evaluation.
- Sharing lessons learned.

Evaluation can help you make sure that your policy is being implemented as planned and that it is having its intended effect. Specifically, evaluation can be used to:
- Identify both barriers to implementing the policy and facilitators of implementation.
- Help improve the rate of compliance with the policy.
- Monitor differences in sub-populations to ensure health equity.
- Demonstrate the value (in terms of impact and effectiveness) and costs of the policy.
- Plan the next steps for implementing the policy and inform future decision making.

Monitoring and Evaluation

Depending on how you will ensure compliance with the policy, resources may be needed for monitoring. For example, one useful resource could be nutritional analysis software. However, if you want each department to have access to this software, allowing each to enter data about its products and menus on its own computer, you may need to purchase more than one license. In addition, consider whether you want to provide training to your staff or contractors on how to use the software.

You will also need resources for evaluation. The evaluations can be conducted in-house, if sufficient staff is available, or by an outside agency, such as a contractor that performs evaluations or an academic institution. An evaluation will help determine whether the initial goals and expected outcomes are being met. It is important to consider evaluation during the planning stage. To look at changes over time, you need to have a baseline measurement (which shows the level of interest before the policy is implemented). Some of the information gathered during the needs assessment stage may be helpful in planning and developing your evaluation plan (see Appendix C for a checklist of key considerations throughout the policy planning process).

When focusing on what types of questions you want to answer in your evaluation, it is important to consider the needs of your stakeholders in this process (e.g., the people or organizations that have an investment in what will be learned from the evaluation and what will be done with results). The types of questions you may want to answer include:

- To what extent have departments implemented the standards?
  - What additional training, resources, and support do departments need to implement the standards more fully?
- What is the impact of the policy?
  - How does it affect the cost of certain foods?
  - How does it affect food or nutrients (such as sodium) that clients consume?
  - How does it affect client health indicators (e.g., blood pressure, weight)?
- Are there any negative or unintended effects of the policy (e.g., fewer people purchasing food from the cafeteria)?
- What does the policy cost to implement (including the costs of staffing, food, etc.)?
  - How do these costs compare to the benefits of the policy?
- What other policies, environmental changes, or interventions can be implemented to increase the impact or support the effectiveness of the food policy?

The methods you use to evaluate your program will depend on the purpose of the evaluation and the types of questions you want to answer. Methods you may want to consider include:

- Collecting data on (or keeping track of) the levels of nutrients of meals served, such as in a nutritional analysis database of the agency's menus.
- Measuring the level of nutrient intake among participants through:
  - Purchase records of products or point-of-purchase surveys.
  - Dietary surveys.
- Measuring changes in the health of participants (e.g., measuring blood pressure or weight).
- Measuring changes in purchase rates and costs (e.g., through records of agency contracts with food vendors or suppliers).
  - Purchase records, including rates of purchase and/or types of purchases.
  - Cost of products and total food budget for each department.
- A record of program costs that includes the time, money, and materials spent to implement the policy.

Sharing Lessons Learned

Once you have been able to implement the procurement policy in your jurisdiction, it is important to share your lessons learned, both the successes and the challenges, with other jurisdictions, including other cities, states, employers, or organizations. Although the experience of each jurisdiction will probably be unique, by letting others know about your experience you can prevent these organizations from having to re-create the wheel. You may want to consider sharing:

- Key steps you undertook to develop and implement the policy.
- Policy language (e.g., what they should make sure is included).

- Challenges you encountered and how you overcame them.
- Cost of implementation.
- Impact.
  - How agencies were able to meet the standards.
  - Changes in participants' intake of nutrients (e.g., of sodium, trans fat, or added sugar).
  - Changes in participants' health outcomes.

You can share your experience through a variety of mechanisms and in different venues, including:
- Success stories or "strategies from the field."
- Tool kit or "how-to" guide.
- Formal report or executive summary.
- Web site or listserv announcement.
- Presentations at professional conferences or regional meetings.
- Peer-reviewed publications.

Sharing your success and lessons learned is a great way to increase the number of settings in your jurisdiction (e.g., private employers, private schools, food programs) that serve healthy meals to consumers. The more settings you can influence, the greater the impact will be!

Appendices

Section Overview:
- Appendix A: Sample Standards.
- Appendix B: Potential Barriers and Solutions.
- Appendix C: Checklist of Key Decisions.

Appendix A: Sample Standards

Appropriate nutrient standards may vary depending on venue. For example, schools may require different nutrient standards than nursing homes would. Some jurisdictions already have procurement standards in place, including New York City, the state of Massachusetts, and, most recently, the U.S. Department of Health and Human Services (HHS). Those standards could be adopted in different jurisdictions if they are appropriate for a specific facility, or new standards could be developed that more adequately suit the particular environment. Some things to consider when deciding whether to draft new standards or to adopt existing standards include:

- Are your food service facilities similar to those that implemented the existing standards?
- Do you have the right resources to implement these standards?
- Are foods available in bulk that could meet these standards?

If you decide to create new standards for your jurisdiction, set up a level that you do not want any food to exceed. In addition, consider such items as components of meals, and think about how much sodium they will have when put together. For example, think of the different components that make up a sandwich, such as bread, meat, and cheese, and consider their individual and collective contributions of sodium and other nutrients.

HHS food standards include minimum standard criteria that all contractors must meet and above-standard criteria that all contractors are encouraged to meet. The HHS food standards require the following for all foods:

- The elimination of partially hydrogenated vegetable oils, shortenings, or margarines for frying, pan-frying (sautéing), grilling, or baking, or as a spread (or for deep frying cake batter and yeast dough), unless the label or other documentation for the oil indicates 0 grams trans fat per serving. Oils and fats used in food preparation and as spreads must also be low in saturated fats. Only foods that are both "0 grams trans fat" and low in saturated fats may be offered.
- All individual food items must contain ≤480 mg sodium as served, and all meals must contain ≤900 mg sodium, as served.

The HHS food standards also include additional requirements related to specific food categories including the following.

Fruits

Standard Criteria:

- All canned or frozen fruits must be packaged in 100% water or unsweetened juice, with no added sweeteners.
- Offer a variety of at least three whole or sliced fruits daily.
- Offer a variety of seasonally available fruits.

Vegetables

Standard Criteria:

- Offer daily at least one raw, salad-type vegetable and at least one steamed, baked, or grilled vegetable, seasoned, without fat or oil.
- All vegetable offerings must contain ≤230 mg sodium, as served.
- Mixed dishes containing vegetables must contain ≤480 mg sodium, as served.
- Offer a variety of seasonally available vegetables.

Above Standard:
- Offer at least one prepared vegetable option with ≤140 mg sodium as served.

Cereals and Grains
Standard Criteria:
- When cereal grains are offered (e.g., rice, bread, pasta), then a whole grain option must be offered for that item as the standard choice.
- All cereal, bread, and pasta offerings must contain ≤230 mg sodium per serving.
- At least 50% of breakfast cereals must contain at least 3g of fiber and less than 10g total sugars per serving.

Above Standard:
- When cereal grains are offered (e.g., rice, bread, pasta), a 100% whole grain option must be offered for that item as the standard choice.
- If cereal is offered, offer at least one cereal with ≤140 mg sodium per serving.

Dairy/Yogurt/Cheese/Fluid Milk
Standard Criteria:
- If milk is offered as a beverage, only offer 2%, 1%, and fat-free fluid milk.
- If cottage cheese items are offered, only offer low fat (2% or less) or fat-free items.
- If yogurt is offered, only offer 2%, 1%, or fat-free yogurt.
- If yogurt is offered, only offer yogurt with no added caloric sweeteners or yogurts labeled as reduced or less sugar according to FDA labeling standards.
- Processed cheeses must contain ≤230 mg sodium per serving.

Protein Foods
Standard Criteria:
- When protein entrees are offered, offer lean meat, poultry, fish, or low-fat vegetarian entrée choices.
- At least twice per week, offer an entrée with a vegetarian protein source.
- Canned or frozen tuna, seafood, and salmon must contain <290 mg sodium per serving, and canned meat <480 mg sodium per serving.

Above Standard:
- A vegetarian entrée must be offered every day.

Beverages
Standard Criteria:
- At least 50% of available beverage choices (other than 100% juice and unsweetened milk) must contain ≤40 calories per serving.
- If juice is offered, only offer 100% juice with no added caloric sweeteners.
- Vegetable juices must contain ≤230 mg sodium per serving.
- Drinking water, preferably chilled tap, must be offered at no charge at all meal service events.

Above Standard:
- For beverages with more than 40 calories per serving, only offer servings of 12 oz or less (excluding unsweetened milk and 100% juice).
- At least 75% of beverage choices (other than 100% juice and unsweetened milk) must contain ≤40 calories per serving.

- Offer as a choice a non-dairy, calcium-fortified beverage (such as soy or almond beverage); these beverages must not provide more sugars than milk (thus must be 12 g sugar per 8 oz serving or less), must provide about the same amount of protein (at least 6 g per 8 oz serving) and calcium (250 mg per 8 oz serving), and must provide less than 5 g total fat (equivalent to 2% milk).
- Offer at least one low-sodium vegetable juice (≤140 mg sodium per serving).

Other Considerations
Standard Criteria:
- Deep-fried options must not be marketed or promoted as the special or feature of the day.
- Limit deep-fried entrée options to no more than one choice per day.
- Offer half- or reduced-size choices for some meals and concession items, when feasible.
- Where value meal combinations are offered, always offer fruit or a non-fried vegetable as the optional side dish, instead of chips or a cookie.

Above Standard:
- Make healthier options more appealing to the consumer by offering them at a reduced price as compared to less healthy alternatives.
- Offer desserts that use less or no added sugars. For example, offer desserts prepared with fruits, vegetables, nuts, seeds, apple sauces, and yogurts without added sugars.

The New York City Agency Food Standards require that no single purchased food item exceed 480 mg of sodium per serving. However, the agency has set stricter standards for food groups (breads, cereals, canned and frozen seafood). These standards may be found at http://www.nyc.gov/html/doh/html/cardio/cardio-vend-nutrition-standard.shtml.

Appendix B: Potential Barriers and Solutions[8]

Barriers	Solutions
Unique features among food service settings **(e.g., prisons vs. day care centers vs. work sites)**	• Involve settings in developing the policy and standards. • Allow different settings to have different standards that are appropriate for the unique features of each setting, including existing food standards, other nutritional mandates, populations served, and current contracts. • Have a different policy or exempt concessioners. • Phase in the standards to demonstrate their feasibility to more reluctant departments. • Maintain a point of contact in each sector to stay abreast of needs that change over time.
Complexity of food service arrangements **(e.g., food served to both staff and patients, existence of multiple grantees or sub-contractors, mandate to work with specific populations such as blind vendors)**	• Allow different settings to implement different standards that meet their needs. • Provide technical assistance or training on how to implement and monitor compliance with standards in different settings. • Condense existing subcontracts into one contract if possible.
Costs and availability of low-sodium foods	• Inquire about current low-sodium options offered by current and potential food service caterers or wholesalers. • Seek vendors who can make available options for sodium that meet the standards. • Allow for benchmark reductions for food items that are particularly difficult to find. • Set up purchasing agreements with other departments and programs to get better prices (bulk purchasing). • Build the capacity of departments (e.g., through "certified purchasing certificates") so they can negotiate lower prices. • Look for currently available and affordable products when developing standards. If needed, make changes to the menu that allow for use of available and affordable options. • Track costs over time. • Increase the proportion of food cooked from scratch (instead of using processed foods) so you can control the amount of sodium that is added to foods. • Solicit donations of healthy foods. • Partner with local farms to get affordable fresh fruits and vegetables. • Partner with other jurisdictions for bulk purchasing.

---

[8] Gase LN, Kuo T, Dunet DO, Simon PA. Facilitators and barriers to implementing a local policy to reduce sodium consumption in the county of Los Angeles government, California, 2009. *Prev Chronic Dis.* 2011;8(2):A33.

	• Perform cost-analysis to demonstrate overall cost-savings in terms of health care costs averted.
Lack of consumer demand for low-sodium foods	• Label and promote healthy items that you offer. For example, use savory descriptors to entice purchase of healthy items, or put a warning symbol on packages containing high-sodium foods. • Subsidize the cost of healthy options or cross-subsidize the prices of healthy and unhealthy options. • Implement public health education campaigns in order to increase awareness, desire, and demand among consumers for healthy options. • Arrange healthy options in highly visible areas and at the point of purchase in cafeterias and other similar venues. • Consider that in some cases consumers won't even notice the change in taste when they are eating a product that is lower in sodium.
Perceptible taste difference between regular- and low-sodium foods	• Make gradual changes to lessen the amount of sodium over time. • Consider how foods "stack up"; a lower-sodium taste may be perceived when consuming an individual product, such as cheese, but it may go undetected when part of a meal, such as lasagna. • Conduct taste tests with target audiences to find the level of sodium reduction that is acceptable; require new items to pass taste tests before they are offered and placed on the menu. • Start by offering healthy options and allowing customers to make a choice about which products to eat (a "healthy foods options" program).
Preference for using prepackaged items	• Cook from scratch (instead of using processed foods) so you can control the amount of sodium that is added to foods; if cooking facilities aren't available, contract with a group that can provide cooking facilities. o If cooking from scratch is not always feasible, consider cooking selected items from scratch. • Enhance refrigeration capacity so that departments can store fresh products for longer periods of time. • Request low-sodium bulk options from the supplier if these same items are available in smaller sizes.
Lack of knowledge and experience in implementing sodium standards	• Provide guidance on how to implement nutrition standards. Respond to individual departments' and audiences' needs (e.g., training cooks on how to prepare low-sodium options). • Provide materials that can be used by different audiences (e.g., precise guidelines on nutrition that could be understood by local food service facilities, approved lists of snacks and supplies). • Connect key points of contact from different sectors (jails and hospitals, for example) so they can learn from each other.
Difficulty modifying existing contracts	• When developing standards, explore what can be done within existing contracts. • Phase in standards so that they take effect the next time the contract is renewed. • Provide standard contract language that departments can use. • Consult with other departments that have been able to modify contracts.

Appendix C: Checklist of Key Decisions

As illustrated by this guide, implementing a food procurement policy can be a large undertaking. To help break down the steps you will need to take, we have included below a checklist of key decisions. This checklist can help you ensure that you have considered all of the necessary steps in the planning, adoption, and implementation phases of a new policy.

Planning

- Do you have the necessary players and departments on board?
- Do you understand which settings the policy will affect?
- Will the policy and nutrition standards work for all the food service settings in your jurisdiction?
- Is the language of the policy specific and clear?
- Have you determined, and secured, the resources needed for implementation of the policy?

Adoption

- Do you understand the process by which the policy will be adopted?
- Have you presented information to the decision makers in a clear, meaningful, and timely way?

Implementation

- Have you identified a point of contact in each of the settings that will implement the policy?
- Have you assessed the training needs of different audiences and delivered appropriate trainings?
- Have you created products and materials for different audiences in order to facilitate implementation?
- Have you created a system to ensure compliance?
- Have you developed an evaluation plan to measure progress?
- How will you share with other entities the lessons you have learned?

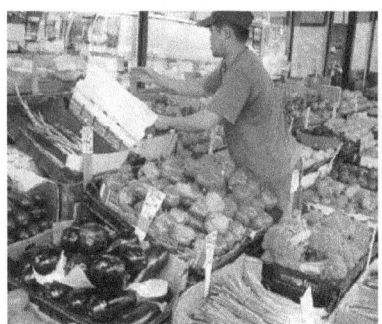 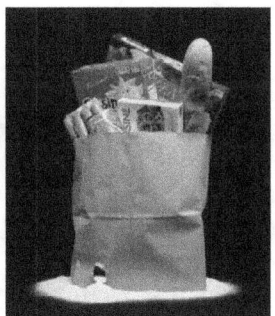 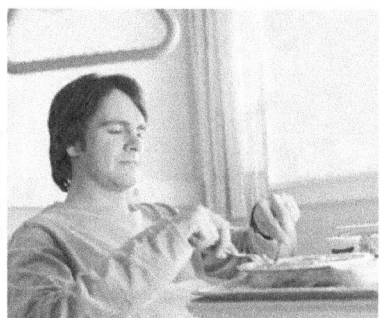 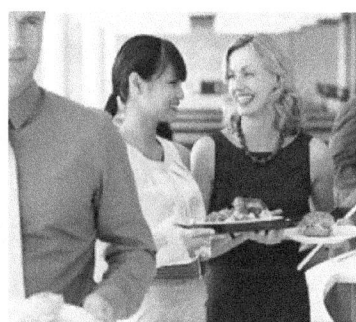

For more information please contact Centers for Disease Control and Prevention
1600 Clifton Road NE, Atlanta, GA 30333
Telephone: 1-800-CDC-INFO (232-4636)/TTY: 1-888-232-6348
E-mail: cdcinfo@cdc.gov
Web: www.cdc.gov